The obesity protocol: "The Revolutionary Plan to Combat Obesity and Reclaim Health"

Dolores E. Flint

Table of Contents

INTRODUCTION

Obesity has recently emerged as one of the world's most significant public health issues. It was once thought to be a problem, particularly in rich countries, but it has now spread worldwide, affecting people of various ages, socioeconomic backgrounds, and ethnicities. Understanding the multidimensional nature of obesity is critical for developing effective methods to combat its prevalence and effects on individuals and societies. This introduction will present a complete review of the obesity epidemic, including its causes, repercussions, and far-reaching ramifications. We will investigate the intricate interplay of genetic, environmental, social, and behavioral factors that contribute to the development and maintenance of obesity. First, we'll look at the distinguishing characteristics of obesity, looking beyond just physical weight to understand the physiological and metabolic changes that occur within the body. Obesity has a significant impact on nearly every system in the human body, from increased adipose tissue accumulation to changes in hormone regulation and inflammatory processes, predisposing people to a variety of chronic health conditions such as type 2 diabetes, cardiovascular disease, certain cancers, and musculoskeletal disorders. Next, we'll look at the underlying reasons for the obesity pandemic, realizing that it's more than just human decision or willpower, but rather a complex mix of hereditary predisposition and environmental factors. Sedentary lifestyles, easy access to high-calorie, nutrient-poor foods, social inequities, cultural norms, and constructed surroundings that discourage physical activity all contribute to the world's rising obesity rate. Furthermore, we will explore the socioeconomic and health inequities associated with obesity, emphasizing the disproportionate impact on disadvantaged communities and underserved populations. From restricted availability of healthy foods and safe recreational areas to discrepancies in healthcare access and quality, socioeconomic factors influence obesity patterns and health outcomes. Furthermore, we will investigate the social consequences of obesity, both in terms of healthcare costs and lost productivity, underlining the critical need for comprehensive prevention and management solutions to combat this epidemic. Understanding the far-reaching consequences of obesity for individuals, families, communities, and societies as a whole helps us comprehend the urgency of taking proactive steps to address this public health epidemic.

Finally, this introduction lays the groundwork for a more in-depth investigation of the obesity pandemic and the numerous measures required to effectively tackle it. Recognizing the complex interplay of factors that contribute to obesity and its profound impact on health and well-being allows us to begin developing comprehensive methods that encourage healthy lifestyles, equal access to resources, and supportive settings conducive to long-term health and vitality.

Chapter 1: The Science of Obesity: Causes and Consequences

Obesity is a complicated disorder influenced by a variety of biological, environmental, and behavioral factors, rather than just being the result of overeating or a lack of willpower. In this chapter, we will delve into the complex science of obesity, investigating its fundamental origins and its far-reaching effects on human health.

1. **Genetic Predisposition:** While genetics do not dictate an individual's risk of obesity, they do play an important role in predisposing people to weight increase and adiposity. Certain genetic variants can influence metabolism, appetite management, and fat accumulation, rendering some people more prone to obesity than others.

2. **Environmental Factors:** The modern environment is full of obesogenic stimuli that encourage binge eating and sedentary behavior. Easy access to high-calorie, nutrient-poor foods, along with omnipresent advertising and food marketing, can result in excessive calorie consumption. Furthermore, sedentary lifestyles caused by technology improvements, urbanization, and changes in transportation and work habits all lead to lower energy expenditure and higher obesity rates.

3. **Hormonal Imbalance:** Hormones control hunger, metabolism, and fat accumulation. Imbalances in hormones such as leptin, insulin, ghrelin, and cortisol can impair the body's capacity to maintain energy balance, resulting in increased food intake, decreased satiety, and altered fat storage.

4. **Neurobiological Factors:** The brain controls food intake and energy expenditure via various neurobiological mechanisms. Dysregulation of neurotransmitters and reward circuits in the brain can cause compulsive overeating and addictive behaviors, which contribute to obesity development.

5. **Socioeconomic Factors:** Socioeconomic status increases obesity risk by affecting the availability of healthful meals, opportunities for physical activity, and exposure to chronic stresses. Individuals from lower socioeconomic origins frequently encounter challenges such as food instability, restricted access to healthcare, and a lack of secure recreational spaces in their neighborhoods, worsening their obesity risk.

Obesity-related consequences:

1. **Chronic Health Conditions:** Obesity is a major risk factor for a wide range of chronic health issues, including type 2 diabetes, cardiovascular disease, hypertension, dyslipidemia, some malignancies, and musculoskeletal diseases. These conditions have a substantial influence on quality of life and raise the chance of premature death.

2. **Psychological Impact:** Obesity can have serious psychological consequences, such as low self-esteem, sadness, anxiety, and body image dissatisfaction. Individuals with obesity have additional mental health issues due to stigma and discrimination, making it difficult to seek help and engage in healthy activities.

3. **Economic Burden:** Obesity imposes significant economic costs on people, healthcare institutions, and society as a whole. Obesity-related medical treatment incurs large direct and indirect expenses, including missed productivity and incapacity, putting a burden on healthcare resources and impeding socio-economic growth.

In conclusion, obesity is a complicated and multifaceted disorder with far-reaching implications for individual health, society's well-being, and healthcare systems. Understanding the fundamental science of obesity and its various causes and implications allows us to develop more effective prevention, intervention, and treatment techniques, ultimately leading to a healthier and more equitable future for all.

Chapter 2: Assessing Your Health and Identifying Risk Factors

Before embarking on any health journey, you must first examine your existing health status and identify potential risk factors for obesity and related chronic conditions. In this chapter, we will look at different ways to assess health and identify the risk factors connected with obesity.

1. **Body Mass Index (BMI):** BMI is a widely used metric that compares body weight to height and divides people into weight groups such as underweight, normal weight, overweight, and obese. While BMI is a valuable screening tool, it has limitations and does not consider muscle mass or body composition.

2. **Waist Circumference:** Abdominal obesity, defined as a larger waist circumference, is a major risk factor for obesity-related health problems such as cardiovascular disease, type 2 diabetes, and metabolic syndrome. Waist circumference measurement, when combined with BMI, can assist in identifying those who are more likely to develop these illnesses.

3. **Body Composition Analysis:** Measuring body composition, including the distribution of lean and fat mass, provides a more complete picture of one's health than BMI alone. Dual-energy X-ray absorptiometry (DEXA), bioelectrical impedance analysis (BIA), and underwater weighing are all methods for determining body fat percentage and identifying persons with excess adiposity.

4. **Family History:** Genetic predisposition is a crucial factor in obesity risk, with family history serving as an essential predictor of sensitivity to weight increase and accompanying health issues. Individuals who have a family history of obesity, type 2 diabetes, cardiovascular disease, or other metabolic diseases may be at a higher risk and should closely monitor their health.

5. **Lifestyle Factors:** Examining lifestyle habits such as food patterns, physical activity levels, sleep quality, stress management, and tobacco or alcohol use can help identify potential risk factors for obesity and chronic disease development. Unhealthy lifestyle habits, such as sedentary behavior, poor eating choices, and insufficient sleep, can all lead to weight gain and metabolic abnormalities.

6. **Metabolic Health Markers:** Monitoring metabolic health markers such as blood pressure, blood glucose levels, lipid profile (e.g., cholesterol and triglycerides), and inflammatory markers (e.g., C-reactive protein) can assist in identifying individuals at risk for obesity-related complications such as hypertension, insulin resistance, dyslipidemia, and inflammation.

7. **Psychological Factors:** Stress, depression, emotional eating, and disordered eating patterns can all affect weight management behaviors and increase the risk of obesity. Assessing psychological well-being and addressing underlying mental health difficulties are critical components of comprehensive obesity prevention and control strategies.

By carefully analyzing your health and recognizing potential risk factors for obesity and related chronic diseases, you can make proactive efforts to reduce risk, adopt healthier lifestyle habits, and seek appropriate medical advice as needed. Remember that prevention and early intervention are essential for preserving good health and well-being throughout life.

Chapter 3: The Obesity Protocol Unveiled: A Step-by-Step Guide.

Without a clear road map, embarking on a journey toward healthy weight management and general well-being can be intimidating. In this chapter, we introduce the Obesity Protocol, a thorough step-by-step program that enables people to take charge of their health and achieve long-term weight loss success.

1. **Setting Clear Goals:** To begin your weight loss journey, set clear and realistic goals. Consider both short- and long-term goals, and ensure they are precise, measurable, attainable, relevant, and time-bound (SMART). Having specific goals, such as decreasing a certain amount of pounds, improving metabolic indicators, or increasing overall fitness, will help you stay focused and motivated.

2. **Assessing preparedness for Change:** Consider your preparedness for change and willingness to commit to healthy lifestyle choices. Evaluate your readiness in several areas, including nutrition, physical exercise, stress management, sleep hygiene, and social support. Recognize any limitations or difficulties that may hamper your success and devise tactics to overcome them.

3. **Creating a Personalized strategy:** Consult with a healthcare specialist or competent professional to develop a strategy that is tailored to your specific needs, preferences, and health state. Your strategy should include dietary changes, physical exercise guidelines, behavior modification tactics, and any necessary medical measures. When creating your strategy, take into account your food preferences, cultural background, medical history, and lifestyle limits.

4. **Adopting a Balanced Diet:** Aim for a balanced and nutritious diet that includes whole, minimally processed foods including fruits, vegetables, lean proteins, whole grains, and healthy fats. Use portion control, mindful eating, and moderation when making food choices, and limit your intake of highly processed, sugary, and calorie-dense foods that contribute to weight gain and metabolic dysfunction.

5. **Incorporating Regular Physical Activity:** Try to incorporate regular physical activity into your daily routine, including both aerobic and strength training. Choose activities that you enjoy and can sustain over time, such as walking, cycling, swimming, dancing, or group fitness programs. Aim for at least 150 minutes of moderate-intensity aerobic activity or 75 minutes of vigorous-intensity aerobic activity per week, with muscle-strengthening activities on two or more days.

6. **Using Behavioral Strategies:** To help you lose weight, set SMART goals, track your food intake and physical activity, identify overeating triggers, practice stress management techniques, cultivate a supportive social network, and celebrate small victories along the way. Create coping mechanisms to deal with cravings,

emotional eating, and setbacks, and seek help from
friends, family, or a support group as needed.

7. **Monitoring Progress and Adjusting methods:**
Regularly track your progress toward your goals and
alter your methods in response to feedback from your
body and your healthcare team. Keep track of your
weight, body measurements, food intake, physical
activity levels, and other important data to monitor your
improvement over time. Be adaptable and willing to
change your approach as needed to overcome plateaus,
handle problems, and ensure long-term success.

By following the Obesity Protocol step by step, you can
achieve long-term weight loss and better health
outcomes. Remember that everyone's path to wellness
is unique, so listen to your body, seek help when
necessary, and approach your journey with patience,
tenacity, and self-compassion.

Chapter 4: Nutrition Essentials: Fueling Your Body for Maximum Health

Nutrition is critical in promoting overall health and well-
being, regulating everything from energy levels and
metabolism to immune function and illness prevention.

In this chapter, we'll look at the fundamental principles of nutrition and offer practical advice for nourishing your body for optimal health.

1. **Balanced Macronutrients:** A balanced diet contains a variety of macronutrients—carbohydrates, proteins, and fats—in the proper quantities to meet your body's energy requirements and support numerous physiological activities. Consume a range of nutrient-dense foods high in complex carbs, lean proteins, and healthy fats to offer long-term energy and encourage satiety.

2. **Entire Foods vs. Processed Foods:** Choose entire, less processed foods over highly processed, refined products wherever feasible. Fruits, vegetables, whole grains, legumes, nuts, seeds, lean meats, and fish are high in vitamins, minerals, fiber, and phytonutrients, whereas processed meals frequently have added sugars, bad fats, sodium, and artificial additives, all of which can hurt health.

3. **Portion Control and Mindful Eating:** Use portion control and mindful eating to avoid overeating and increase your awareness of hunger and fullness cues. Pay attention to your body's hunger and satiety cues, eat deliberately, taste every meal, and avoid distractions like television or screens when eating. Using smaller dishes, bowls, and utensils can also help with portion control.

4. **Hydration:** Stay well-hydrated by drinking enough water throughout the day. Water is required to regulate body temperature, facilitate nutrition transport, aid digestion, and eliminate toxins from the body. Aim to

consume at least 8-10 cups of water every day, or more if you are physically active or in hot weather.

5. **Nutrient Density:** Choose meals that are high in key nutrients and offer the best nutritious value for your money. Nutrient-dense foods including leafy greens, colorful vegetables, berries, nuts, seeds, whole grains, lean meats, and fatty fish are high in vitamins, minerals, antioxidants, and phytonutrients, which promote good health and lower the risk of chronic diseases.

6. **Meal Planning and Preparation:** Plan and prepare meals ahead of time to ensure that you have healthful options on hand throughout the week. Batch cooking, meal preparation, and creative leftover use can all help save time and make healthy eating more practical and doable, even on the busiest days. Each meal should contain a range of colorful fruits and vegetables, fiber-rich carbs, healthy fats, and a balance of protein.

7. **Individualized Approach:** Recognize that nutrition is not one-size-fits-all and that individual requirements may differ depending on age, gender, activity level, metabolic rate, health state, and dietary preferences. Experiment with various meals, meal patterns, and eating methods to see what works best for you and helps you achieve your specific health objectives.

Prioritizing nutrition needs and eating a balanced, whole-foods-based diet can help you fuel your body for maximum health, vigor, and longevity. Remember to pay attention to your body's hunger and fullness cues, and approach eating with awareness, enjoyment, and thankfulness for the sustenance it gives.

Chapter 5: Exercise Programs for Weight Management and Overall Health

Regular physical activity is critical for maintaining a healthy weight, improving overall health, and lowering the risk of chronic diseases. In this chapter, we'll look at different workout regimes that are designed for weight management and overall wellness.

Cardiovascular exercises:

• Moderate-intensity cardio: Activities like brisk walking, cycling, swimming, and dancing raise your heart rate and burn calories. Aim for at least 150 minutes of moderate-intensity cardio every week, or 75 minutes of vigorous-intensity cardio for even better results.

• High-intensity Interval Training (HIIT): HIIT consists of short bursts of vigorous exercise followed by rest or low-intensity activities. HIIT workouts are an efficient and effective way to burn calories, improve cardiovascular fitness, and raise metabolism.

Strength Training:

• Resistance Exercises: Strength training with body weight, free weights, resistance bands, or weight machines promotes lean muscle mass, increases metabolic rate, and improves overall strength and endurance. Aim to include resistance exercises targeting key muscle groups at least twice a week.

• Progressive Overload: Gradually increase the intensity, duration, or resistance of your strength training routines over time to keep your muscles challenged while also encouraging muscle growth and adaptation.

Flexibility and Mobility Training:

• **Stretching Exercises:** Use stretching exercises to increase flexibility, mobility, and range of motion in your joints and muscles. Perform dynamic stretches before exercise to warm up your body, and static stretches after exercise to cool down and relax.

• **Yoga or Pilates:** Yoga and Pilates use stretching, strengthening, and mindfulness exercises to improve flexibility, core stability, and mind-body awareness.

Functional training:

• **Functional Exercises:** Functional training focuses on movements that are similar to regular tasks to improve total functional fitness and mobility patterns. Squats, lunges, push-ups, and planks work for several muscular groups while improving balance, coordination, and proprioception.

• **Balance and Stability Training:** Use balance and stability exercises like single-leg stands, balance boards, and stability balls to improve proprioception, lower the chance of falling, and increase total functional capacity.

Mind/Body Practices:

• **Mindfulness and Meditation:** Include mindfulness and meditation activities in your exercise routine to reduce stress, improve mental clarity, and boost general well-being. Tai chi, qigong, and mindful walking are examples of mindful movement practices that combine physical activity and mindfulness techniques to promote relaxation and stress reduction.

• **Breathing Exercises:** Deep breathing techniques can help soothe the nervous system, boost oxygen flow to muscles, and improve relaxation and recuperation after activity.

Consistency and variety:

• **Consistency:** Make exercise a part of your daily routine by scheduling and prioritizing it like any other key obligation.

• **Range:** Make your workouts interesting and challenging by incorporating a range of exercises, activities, and training methods that target different muscle groups, minimize boredom, and prevent overuse problems.

A balanced exercise plan that combines cardiovascular, strength, flexibility, and mind-body training will help you control your weight, increase your overall fitness, and improve your quality of life. Remember to listen to your body, go at your own pace, and get advice from a competent fitness professional if necessary to ensure safe and effective exercise programming.

Chapter 6: Mental Health and Obesity: Addressing Psychological Factors

Mental health and obesity have a complicated and bidirectional relationship, with psychological factors having an important role in obesity development, maintenance, and management. In this chapter, we will look at the psychological elements of obesity and how to handle them effectively.

Emotional Eating & Stress:

• **Emotional Triggers:** Emotional eating, which involves consuming food in response to emotions rather than hunger, is a frequent coping method for stress, worry, melancholy, boredom, and other negative feelings. Recognize emotional triggers for overeating and devise alternate coping mechanisms, such as practicing relaxation techniques, finding social support, or engaging in fun hobbies.

• **Stress Management:** Chronic stress can lead to weight gain and obesity by influencing appetite regulation, cravings for high-calorie meals, and metabolic changes. Deep breathing, mindfulness meditation, yoga, or progressive muscle relaxation are all stress management practices that can help you lower your stress and improve your eating habits.

Body image and self-esteem:

• **Body Dissatisfaction:** Obese people frequently have negative body image and low self-esteem, which can lead to feelings of shame, guilt, and low self-worth. Challenge negative body image attitudes and develop self-compassion and acceptance for your body at any size.

• **Focus on Health:** Move away from weight-centric goals and toward health-centric goals, emphasizing increases in physical fitness, energy levels, mood, and general well-being. Instead of focusing primarily on weight loss, celebrate non-scale achievements and praise progress toward health-promoting activities.

Cognitive factors:

• **Cognitive Distortions:** Address cognitive distortions or negative thought patterns about food, weight, and body image, such as all-or-nothing thinking, catastrophizing, or categorizing foods as "good" or "bad." Use cognitive restructuring approaches to challenge and reframe erroneous beliefs, resulting in more balanced and adaptable thinking patterns.

• **Mindful Eating:** Use mindful eating strategies to improve your awareness of hunger and satiety cues, enjoy the sensory experience of eating, and create a nonjudgmental attitude toward food and eating behaviors. Slow down, chew your food fully, and pay close attention to the flavor, texture, and level of satisfaction in each bite.

Social Support and Connections:

• **Social Isolation:** Social isolation and a lack of social support can worsen emotions of loneliness, sadness, and emotional eating. Seek help from friends, family, support groups, or mental health experts to connect with others who understand your challenges and can offer encouragement, understanding, and practical advice.

• **Accountability and Encouragement:** Work with a friend, family member, or health coach to provide accountability, motivation, and encouragement during your weight loss journey. Share your objectives, celebrate victories, and work together to keep on track and make long-term growth.

Professional support:

• **Therapy and Counseling:** Consult a licensed mental health practitioner, such as a psychologist, counselor, or therapist, to address underlying emotional difficulties, dysfunctional coping methods, and psychological hurdles to weight loss. Cognitive-behavioral therapy (CBT) and dialectical behavior therapy (DBT) are evidence-based methods for dealing with emotional eating and improving body image.

• **Integrated Care:** Choose integrated care models that address both physical and mental health requirements simultaneously, such as multidisciplinary weight management programs that involve medical, dietary, exercise, and psychological interventions suited to individual needs.

Individuals who address psychological factors such as emotional eating, stress management, body image, cognitive distortions, social support, and professional guidance can cultivate a healthy mindset, develop sustainable lifestyle habits, and attain long-term success with weight management and overall well-being.

Remember that requesting help is a sign of strength, and you do not have to face this path alone.

Chapter 7: Overcoming Challenges: Strategies for Long-Term Success.

Sustaining weight reduction and developing good lifestyle habits over time might be difficult, but with the appropriate tactics and mentality, it is possible. In this chapter, we'll look at crucial techniques for overcoming frequent hurdles and attaining long-term success in your weight loss journey.

Set realistic expectations:

• **Avoid fast remedies:** Recognize that long-term weight loss requires time and work, with no shortcuts or fast remedies. Set reasonable goals for yourself and prioritize making incremental, long-term improvements to your living patterns above achieving quick results.

Enhance Resilience:

• **Mentality Shift:** Adopt a growth mentality and see setbacks and problems as chances for learning and progress, not reasons to give up. Cultivate resilience by viewing setbacks as temporary hurdles and concentrating on solutions and progress rather than lingering on failures.

• **Learn from Mistakes:** Consider your past experiences and find lessons from previous weight loss attempts or obstacles. Use this knowledge to fine-tune your approach, establish more realistic goals, and devise solutions for overcoming future challenges.

Create a Support Network:

• **Seek Support:** Surround yourself with a network of friends, family members, or peers who share your goals and can offer encouragement, accountability, and practical aid. Share your accomplishments and problems with your support group, and celebrate your progress together.

• **Join a Community:** Consider joining a weight loss support group, an online community, or a fitness class where you can meet like-minded people, exchange experiences, and get advice and motivation from others on the same road.

Practice self-compassion:

• **Be Kind to Yourself:** Practice self-compassion and treat yourself with love and empathy, especially when you are struggling or experiencing a setback. Avoid self-criticism and negative self-talk, and instead, treat yourself with the same care and compassion as you would a friend facing comparable circumstances.

• **Prioritize Progress:** Celebrate your accomplishments and progress, no matter how modest, and recognize your efforts and dedication to your health and well-being. Remember that every step forward, no matter how tiny, gets you closer to your goals.

Adaptability & Flexibility:

• **Maintain Flexibility:** Be willing to adjust your approach and modify your goals or strategies as circumstances, preferences, or problems change along the road. Accept flexibility and openness to new ideas, strategies, and solutions that may better meet your changing demands.

• **Prepare for difficulties:** Anticipate any difficulties or barriers that may arise during your weight loss journey, such as holidays, vacations, social gatherings, or periods of elevated stress, and devise contingency plans or coping skills to efficiently traverse these challenges.

Concentrate on Non-Scale Victories:

• **Recognize Progress:** Rather than focusing on the number on the scale, recognize non-scale successes such as increased energy, fitness, mood, sleep quality, clothes fit, or overall quality of life. Recognize and appreciate the good improvements that emerge from your healthy lifestyle choices.

Remain Committed to Long-Term Health:

• **Lifestyle, Not a Diet:** Instead of dieting for a short period, adopt long-term lifestyle behaviors that promote health and wellness. Accept the journey as a lifelong commitment to self-care, prioritizing health and vitality over short-term weight loss goals.

By applying these tactics for overcoming hurdles and maintaining long-term success, you will be able to stay motivated and accomplish long-term weight loss and improved health results. Remember that growth is not linear, and setbacks are a normal part of the process. Stay resilient, motivated, and dedicated to your goals for a healthier, happier future.

Chapter 8: Lifestyle Changes for Sustainable Weight Loss

Weight loss and maintenance involve more than just short-term diets; they also necessitate long-term lifestyle changes that promote healthy habits. In this chapter, we'll look at how to make crucial lifestyle changes for long-term weight loss.

Nutrition Education and Behavioral Change:

• **Balanced Diet:** Eat a variety of full, nutrient-dense foods, including fruits, vegetables, lean meats, whole grains, and healthy fats. Instead of restricting yourself, focus on portion control, mindful eating, and moderation.

• **Nutrition Education:** Learn about macronutrients, micronutrients, food labeling, portion proportions, and mindful eating techniques. Understanding the nutritional value of foods can help you make informed decisions and maintain a positive connection with food.

• **Behavior Change Strategies:** Use behavior modification approaches such as goal setting, self-monitoring, stimulus management, problem-solving, and social support to build and maintain healthy eating habits. Identify triggers for bad eating habits and devise tactics to overcome them.

Physical activity and exercises:

• **Regular Exercise:** Incorporate physical activity into your daily routine to burn calories, enhance cardiovascular health, gain muscle mass, and increase metabolism. Aim for at least 150 minutes of moderate-intensity aerobic exercise or 75 minutes of vigorous-intensity exercise per week, with muscle-strengthening activities on two or more days.

• **Find Enjoyable Activities:** Choose activities that you enjoy and can stick with long-term, such as walking, jogging, cycling, swimming, dancing, or doing group fitness classes. Vary your routines to avoid boredom and target different muscle regions.

• **Lifestyle Integration:** Incorporate physical exercise into your daily life by using active transportation, walking the stairs instead of the elevator, gardening, doing housework, or playing sports with friends and family. Look for opportunities to exercise more during the day, especially if you work in a sedentary environment.

Stress Management & Self-Care:

• **Stress Reduction Techniques:** Deep breathing, meditation, yoga, progressive muscle relaxation, or mindfulness can all help you reduce stress and avoid emotional eating.

• **Self-Care Practices:** Prioritize self-care activities that promote relaxation, rejuvenation, and mental well-being, such as obtaining enough sleep, spending time outside, pursuing hobbies, socializing with loved ones, and indulging in creative activities.

Sleep Hygiene and Restful Sleep:

• **Healthy Sleep Habits:** Make proper sleep hygiene a top priority to guarantee restorative and quality sleep every night. Maintain a consistent sleep schedule, develop a calming bedtime routine, limit screen time before bed, and establish a restful sleep environment.

• **The Role of Sleep in Weight Management:** Recognize the significance of appropriate sleep in regulating hunger hormones, metabolism, energy balance, and food cravings. Aim for 7-9 hours of quality sleep per night to help your weight loss and general health.

Behavioral Monitoring and Accountability:

• **Self-monitoring:** Keep track of your eating patterns, physical activity levels, and weight loss progress with a notebook, mobile app, or wearable activity tracker. Self-monitoring encourages awareness, accountability, and the recognition of patterns and trends.

• **Accountability Partners:** Work with a friend, family member, or support group to provide accountability, motivation, and encouragement during your weight loss journey. To keep on track and sustain momentum, share your goals, recognize victories, and collaborate to overcome obstacles.

You can achieve long-term weight loss and enhance your overall health and well-being by making lifestyle changes that prioritize nutrition, physical activity, stress management, sleep hygiene, and behavior change. Remember that little, consistent improvements over time can lead to major and long-term outcomes, and aim for progress rather than perfection on your path to a healthier lifestyle.

Chapter 9: Understanding Social and Environmental Influences

Social and environmental factors influence our food patterns, physical activity levels, and general lifestyle choices. Navigating these factors skillfully is critical for developing healthy behaviors and achieving long-term weight management success. This chapter will look at ways to negotiate social and environmental pressures to help you lose weight.

Social support:

• **Surround Yourself with Supportive People:** Create a supportive social network of friends, family members, or peers who understand and respect your health objectives. Surrounding oneself with positive influencers can help you stay motivated, accountable, and on track.

• **Communicate Your Needs:** Be open and honest with your loved ones about your health objectives and the value of their assistance. Communicate your requirements, preferences, and boundaries for food, social activities, and other lifestyle elements that may affect your weight loss journey.

Healthy socializing:

• **Plan Ahead for Social Events:** Anticipate social gatherings, parties, and outings when food and beverages may be plentiful, and prepare to make healthier choices. Consider eating a healthy meal or snack beforehand, bringing a nutritious dish to share, or suggesting non-food-related activities.

• **Practice Assertiveness:** Use assertive communication skills to advocate for your health needs and preferences in social settings. Learn to gracefully decline peer pressure or undesirable temptations, and set boundaries without feeling guilty or forced to conform.

Environmental cues:

• **Create a Supportive Environment:** Design your home and work environments to encourage healthy habits while reducing reasons for overeating or inactive behavior. Stock your kitchen with nutritious foods, have healthy snacks on hand, and eliminate or limit access to harmful temptations.

• **Mindful Eating:** Use mindful eating practices to become more conscious of environmental cues that may influence your eating habits, such as portion sizes, food availability, visual cues, and social effects. Pay attention to your hunger and satiety cues and make informed decisions about when, what, and how much to eat.

Food Environment:

• **Make healthier choices Convenient:** Choose convenience foods that are in line with your health goals by prepping and portioning nutritious meals and snacks ahead of time. Keep healthful grab-and-go items like fruits, vegetables, almonds, and yogurt on hand for quick and simple access.

• **Navigate Food Marketing:** Be wary of food marketing methods and false labeling practices that may encourage unhealthy or decadent foods. Learn how to critically assess food marketing, packaging claims, and restaurant menus so you can make informed decisions that support your health goals.

Social and cultural influences:

• **Respect Cultural Traditions:** Honor your cultural background and traditions while making deliberate choices to promote your health and well-being. Find ways to incorporate cultural foods and practices into your healthy eating plan, as well as to improve the nutritional value of traditional meals.

• **Negotiate Social Norms:** Be confident and forceful when navigating social norms and peer pressure connected to food and eating patterns. Remember that it is acceptable to break from social norms and make decisions that are consistent with your personal values and health goals.

Seek Community Support:

• **Join Supportive Communities:** Look for online or in-person communities, support groups, or weight loss programs where you can interact with people who have similar objectives and struggles. Participating in a supportive group can help you stay motivated, accountable, and encouraged on your weight reduction journey.

By carefully and proactively managing social and environmental forces, you can build a supportive ecosystem that allows you to make better choices, overcome challenges, and achieve long-term weight management success. Remember that you can modify your environment and surroundings to reflect your health objectives and ideals.

Chapter 10: Managing Obesity with Medical Interventions

While lifestyle changes are the foundation of obesity management, medicinal therapies can be extremely beneficial in aiding weight loss attempts, particularly for people with severe obesity or obesity-related comorbidities. In this chapter, we'll look at the many medical strategies available for treating obesity and improving health outcomes.

Pharmacotherapy:

• **Weight Loss drugs:** Prescription drugs approved by regulatory authorities such as the Food and Drug Administration (FDA) may be recommended to aid in weight loss when lifestyle changes alone are insufficient. These drugs act by lowering appetite, limiting meal intake, or preventing fat absorption. Examples include phentermine, liraglutide, orlistat, and naltrexone/bupropion.

• **Combination Therapies:** Certain weight reduction drugs are available in combination formulations to increase efficacy and tolerance. Combination medicines may target various mechanisms involved in appetite regulation and energy metabolism, resulting in improved weight loss outcomes.

• **Patient Selection and Monitoring:** Weight reduction drugs should be provided with caution and adapted to each patient's specific needs, taking into account factors such as obesity severity, comorbidities, medication history, and potential side effects. Regular monitoring and follow-up with a healthcare professional are required to assess therapy response, ensure patient safety, and change prescription regimens as needed.

Bariatric surgeries:

• **Surgical Options:** Bariatric surgery, commonly known as weight reduction surgery, includes a variety of techniques that alter the digestive system to facilitate weight loss and metabolic changes. Gastric bypass, sleeve gastrectomy, adjustable gastric banding, and biliopancreatic diversion with duodenal switch are among the most common bariatric operations.

• **Processes of Action:** Bariatric surgery causes weight reduction through a variety of processes, including reduced food intake, changes in gut hormones involved in appetite regulation and glucose metabolism, and changes in gut microbiota composition.

• **Indications and Eligibility:** Bariatric surgery is advised for persons with severe obesity (BMI > 40 kg/m²) or moderate obesity (BMI ≥ 35 kg/m²) with obesity-related comorbidities who have not achieved significant weight loss through lifestyle therapies or medicines. Eligibility criteria may differ depending on age, BMI, comorbidities, and patient preferences.

Endoscopic interventions:

• **Minimally Invasive Procedures:** Endoscopic procedures are less invasive alternatives to traditional bariatric surgery and may be appropriate for people who want to lose weight without having surgery. Gastric balloon implantation, endoscopic sleeve gastroplasty, or gastric artery embolization are all operations that use an endoscope to access and treat the gastrointestinal tract.

• **Safety and efficacy:** Endoscopic interventions are typically regarded as safe and well-tolerated, with fewer risks and consequences than surgical procedures. However, its efficacy for long-term weight loss may be limited, and long-term evidence on outcomes is still in the early stages.

Complete Multidisciplinary Care:

• **Integrated Approach:** Effective obesity management frequently necessitates teamwork among healthcare specialists from multiple disciplines, such as physicians, dietitians, psychologists, exercise physiologists, and bariatric surgeons. A comprehensive care paradigm tackles not only weight loss, but also linked comorbidities, psychosocial problems, and obesity-related behaviors.

• **Individualized Treatment Plans:** Tailoring therapies to individual patient's needs and preferences is crucial for improving outcomes and encouraging long-term adherence to treatment recommendations. Personalized treatment regimens may include a combination of lifestyle changes, medicinal therapy, behavioral counseling, and surgical procedures, depending on the patient's characteristics and goals.

Ongoing Monitoring and Support:

• **Long-Term Follow-Up:** Obesity management requires regular monitoring and follow-up care to assess progress, resolve difficulties, and give ongoing support and direction. Throughout the treatment process, healthcare personnel play an important role in monitoring weight loss trajectories, analyzing metabolic parameters, managing medication regimens, and addressing psychosocial concerns.

• **Lifestyle Maintenance:** Helping patients maintain healthy lifestyle practices after the first weight reduction phase is crucial for preventing weight regain and ensuring long-term success. Lifestyle maintenance strategies might involve ongoing nutritional counseling, physical activity promotion, behavior change tactics, and psychosocial support.

Finally, medical therapies play an important role in obesity management by giving extra tools and resources to help people lose weight and improve their health. Individual patient characteristics, preferences, and treatment goals should, however, guide the selection of appropriate interventions, with a focus on personalized, comprehensive care that addresses the complex interplay of biological, behavioral, and environmental factors contributing to obesity.

Chapter 11: Success Story: Real-Life Transformations

Real-life success stories can provide great inspiration and encouragement for people starting their weight loss journeys. These tales show that effort, perseverance, and support can lead to long-term weight loss and health transformation. In this chapter, we'll look at a few encouraging success stories from people who have battled obesity and improved their lives.

Sarah's journey:

• **Starting Point:** Sarah has struggled with obesity since she was a youngster, resulting in a variety of health difficulties and low self-esteem. She weighed more than 300 pounds at her heaviest and felt imprisoned in a cycle of poor eating habits and sedentary behavior.

• **Turning Point:** Determined to regain control of her health, Sarah set out on a voyage of self-discovery and transformation. She got help from a certified dietitian and a therapist to address her emotional eating habits and establish healthy coping methods.

• **Transformation:** With constant work and commitment, Sarah established a balanced diet high in whole foods and focused on regular physical activity, progressively raising her fitness level over time. She shed more than 150 pounds and rediscovered her confidence, energy, and enthusiasm for life.

• **Maintaining Success:** Sarah continues to put her health first by being active, eating mindfully, and seeking support from her community and loved ones. She now serves as an inspiration to others going through similar hardships, sharing her story to inspire and empower them on their paths.

John's Transformation:

• **Beginning Point:** John has struggled with weight and obesity-related health conditions for the majority of his adult life, including type 2 diabetes, high blood pressure, and joint discomfort. He felt imprisoned in a cycle of yo-yo diets and unsuccessful weight loss attempts.

* **Tipping Point:** After a health scare landed him in the hospital, John realized he needed to make major adjustments to enhance his health and quality of life. He sought advice from a multidisciplinary team of healthcare professionals, which included a physician, dietician, and exercise physiologist.

* **Transformation:** With the help of his healthcare team, John established long-term lifestyle changes like as eating a balanced diet, getting more physical activity, and focusing on stress management and sleep hygiene. He shed more than 100 pounds and effectively corrected his diabetes and other metabolic issues.

* **Maintaining Success:** John prioritizes his health by staying active, watching his food, and getting frequent check-ups from his healthcare team. He has accepted his new lifestyle with thankfulness and commitment, knowing that his hard work has resulted in better health and longevity.

Maria's Inspirational Journey:

• **Beginning Point:** Maria suffered from obesity and emotional eating for years, utilizing food as a source of comfort and a coping technique for stress and worry. She was ashamed of her figure and avoided social situations and activities she had previously enjoyed.

• **Tipping Point:** Motivated by a friend's success story, Maria resolved to take control of her health and break free from the cycle of emotional eating. She got help from a therapist who specialized in cognitive-behavioral therapy (CBT) and joined a weight loss support group for accountability and motivation.

• **Transformation:** Through therapy, self-reflection, and peer support, Maria was able to identify and question her negative thought patterns, as well as build healthy coping skills for stress and emotions. She progressively developed a more balanced eating style and recovered control of her health and well-being.

• **Maintaining Success:** Maria prioritizes her emotional and physical health by practicing self-care, setting boundaries, and remaining in touch with her support system. She now lives her life with increased confidence and resilience, seeing setbacks as chances for growth and self-development.

These success stories serve as compelling reminders that transformation is possible at any age, and that failures are not permanent hurdles, but rather opportunities for learning and progress. By sharing their stories, these people instill hope and empower others to trust in themselves and their potential to overcome adversity and reach their health objectives.

Chapter 12: Maintaining Progress: Strategies for Weight Management

Weight loss is a big accomplishment, but maintaining that success over time can be just as difficult. To ensure that your hard-earned results last, you must apply tactics designed exclusively for weight maintenance. In this chapter, we'll look at crucial measures for maintaining progress and avoiding weight regain.

Lead a Balanced Lifestyle:

• **Consistency is Key:** Stick to the healthy habits and behaviors that helped you lose weight, such as frequent physical activity, mindful eating, and appropriate sleep. Consistency in lifestyle practices is essential for avoiding weight return and achieving long-term success.

• **Focus on Health, Not Just Weight:** Instead of focusing just on the number on the scale, consider your entire health and well-being. Emphasize activities that promote good health, such as eating nutrient-dense foods, being active, managing stress, and prioritizing self-care.

Set realistic goals:

• **Maintain a Realistic Weight Range:** Determine a realistic weight maintenance target that is appropriate for your body and lifestyle. Rather than striving for an artificial "ideal" weight, seek to maintain a weight that makes you feel healthy, energized, and at ease in your skin.

• **Focus on Non-Scale Victories:** Celebrate non-scale triumphs, such as gains in fitness, strength, flexibility, energy, mood, and overall quality of life. Recognize and embrace the beneficial changes that occur as a result of your healthy practices, not only weight changes.

Practice Mindful Eating:

• **Listen to Your Body:** Pay attention to your body's hunger and satiety cues, and eat consciously to avoid overeating and increase meal enjoyment. Pay attention to your body's signals of hunger, fullness, and satisfaction, and treat your physical and emotional needs without judgment.

• **Enjoy Your Food:** Eat carefully, relish each bite, and take note of the flavor, texture, and aroma of your meals. Engage all of your senses in the eating experience, and choose foods that you actually like while also nourishing your body and spirit.

Remain Active and Engaged:

• **Find Activities You Enjoy:** Stay physically active by doing something you enjoy, such as walking, cycling, swimming, dancing, hiking, or playing sports. Choose activities that make you happy and fulfilled, and incorporate activity into your everyday routine.

• **Mix It Up:** To keep your workouts interesting and difficult, incorporate a variety of activities and exercises throughout your regimen. Changing up your training routine not only keeps you from becoming bored but also helps you target various muscle areas and avoid overuse issues.

Managing Stress and Emotions:

• **Develop Effective Coping Mechanisms:** Create healthy coping strategies for dealing with stress, emotions, and emotional eating triggers. Deep breathing, meditation, yoga, and journaling are all relaxation activities that can help you reduce stress and improve your mental health.

• **Seek Support:** During stressful or challenging times, seek emotional support and encouragement from friends, family members, or support groups. A robust support network can offer comfort, perspective, and encouragement to help you stay on track with your weight maintenance goals.

Plan and be prepared:

• **Meal Planning:** Plan your meals and snacks ahead of time so that you have healthful options on hand when hunger strikes. Stock your kitchen with nutritious essentials, plan meals ahead of time, and keep portable snacks on hand for busy days or trips.

• **Anticipate Issues:** Consider probable difficulty or triggers for overeating or unhealthy eating patterns, such as social gatherings, holidays, or times of high stress. Create coping methods and contingency plans to efficiently navigate these challenges while remaining on track with your health goals.

Ongoing monitoring and evaluation:

• **Maintain Accountability:** Continue to monitor your progress, actions, and outcomes regularly to keep you accountable and on track with your weight management goals. Keep a diet and activity record, monitor your weight regularly, and evaluate your commitment to healthy practices.

• **Adjust as Needed:** Be adaptable and willing to change your techniques or habits as circumstances, preferences, or goals shift. If you observe indicators of weight regain or lapses in healthy habits, take proactive actions to address them and return to your fitness path.

By using these weight maintenance measures, you may protect your progress, maintain your accomplishments, and live a healthy, full lifestyle for years to come. Remember that making progress is a continual process, and it is natural to experience ups and downs along the road. Be patient, resilient, and committed to your health and well-being.

Conclusion:

Starting a journey to lose weight and improve your health is a powerful act of self-care and empowerment. Throughout this guide, we've looked at a variety of tactics, techniques, and interventions to help you along your transformative journey. Now, as you prepare to take the next steps, it's critical to consider the empowered mentality and actionable ideas that will help you thrive in your health and well-being.

Practice self-compassion:

• Understand that gaining and maintaining a healthy weight is a process with ups and downs. Be gentle to yourself, appreciate your accomplishments, and respond to setbacks with compassion and resilience. You deserve to be loved, respected and supported every step of the way.

Develop Self-awareness:

• Take some time to consider your reasons, values, and health-related goals. Develop self-awareness by paying attention to your body's signals, feelings, and desires, and then make decisions that are consistent with your real self and ambitions for a flourishing existence.

Prioritize Sustainable Habits:

• Focus on developing long-term lifestyle habits that nurture your body, mind, and spirit. Choose nutritious foods, engage in regular physical activity, prioritize sleep and stress management, and cultivate meaningful relationships with others who care about your well-being.

Seek Support and Community:

• You do not have to make this journey alone. Seek help from friends, family, healthcare experts, or online communities who understand and appreciate your health objectives. Surround yourself with positive influences that will motivate, inspire, and empower you to succeed.

Embrace Growth and Resilience:

• Look at challenges and setbacks as chances for growth, learning, and self-development. Embrace resilience by adjusting to change, overcoming hardship, and remaining devoted to your health goals with courage, tenacity, and grace.

Living with Purpose and Joy:

• As you continue on your path to health and well-being, remember to live your life with purpose, passion, and joy. Cultivate thankfulness for the gift of vitality, and treasure each moment as an opportunity to live fully and genuinely.

Empower yourself to thrive in your health and well-being by practicing self-compassion, self-awareness, long-term habits, supportive communities, a growth mindset, and joy-filled living. You have the ability inside yourself to live the lively, satisfying life you deserve. Seize this opportunity, believe in your abilities, and go on the path to a better, happier you.

www.ingramcontent.com/pod-product-compliance
Lightning Source LLC
Chambersburg PA
CBHW070738260726
48660CB00007B/2897